Fabyola Lima Madeira

The power of bibliotherapy

AF190953

Fabyola Lima Madeira

The power of bibliotherapy

Love in the form of stories

ScienciaScripts

Imprint

Any brand names and product names mentioned in this book are subject to trademark, brand or patent protection and are trademarks or registered trademarks of their respective holders. The use of brand names, product names, common names, trade names, product descriptions etc. even without a particular marking in this work is in no way to be construed to mean that such names may be regarded as unrestricted in respect of trademark and brand protection legislation and could thus be used by anyone.

Cover image: www.ingimage.com

This book is a translation from the original published under ISBN 978-613-9-74020-8.

Publisher:
Sciencia Scripts
is a trademark of
Dodo Books Indian Ocean Ltd. and OmniScriptum S.R.L publishing group

120 High Road, East Finchley, London, N2 9ED, United Kingdom
Str. Armeneasca 28/1, office 1, Chisinau MD-2012, Republic of Moldova, Europe
Printed at: see last page
ISBN: 978-620-6-23912-3

Acknowledgements

To my parents for all the love and affection for me and my dedicated siblings, through an upbringing/education for life, always with the intention that we would become worthy and capable people to face the challenges of life.

To my brothers Fernando and Fabrício, for their friendship, laughter, jokes, and for being so different, which provided us with a lot of learning.

To my aunt and godmother Fatima, my second mother, for all
the help and for all
the moments lived since the day of my birth, all thanks would be little
for this dear aunt that I love so much.

To my uncle and also godfather Waldir, for all the support especially in our childhood, always cheering us up and participating in our lives, and for having given me a sweet aunt who also became my godmother, Aunt Elaine.

To all my huge family, from all sides, everyone I understand to be
my family, for teaching me that family is made up of all those we
want, because love is what unites us!

To my husband and best friend, Terence, for being a companion of all hours, for his loving and true way, far or near, his presence in my heart is permanent, a source of joy and gratitude for me.

To all my friends, for teaching me how much more grace, colour, movement and life has when we have friends to share happy or sad moments, knowledge, travel, work, study, party and much more.

To my friend Francisco who helped me in the revision, structuring and finalisation of this book, for always encouraging and stimulating me to share the content of these pages.

To the Storytellers group - DPS, represented by every human being who has ever been
part of it
, for the opportunity of constant learning and personal development
based on love and stories.

Summary

CHAPTER 1	**6**
CHAPTER 2	**11**
CHAPTER 3	**14**
CHAPTER 4	**16**
CHAPTER 5	**20**
CHAPTER 6	**25**
CHAPTER 7	**29**
CHAPTER 8	**35**
CHAPTER 9	**38**
CHAPTER 10	**42**

Presentation

The present work aims to bring to the public a constructive dialogue about bibliotherapy, a subject that arouses much interest due to its simplicity and proven effectiveness. Bibliotherapy, known as the practice of telling stories and giving rise to a therapeutic moment of dialogue, reflection and good humour, causing improvements in the physical and emotional state of people, with or without apparent health problems, has also been widely studied for some time.

Considered a science, because it has a marked presence in universities around the world, with research related to its nuances and forms of application, it is a prominent theme in the academic world. This practice is presented here through an analysis of the content in the scientific literature, but mainly by the knowledge about the subject acquired over the years of experience of the author, as a volunteer in the Storytellers Group.

As a member of the group since its inception in 2011 and coordinator of one of its teams, the author practices bibliotherapeutic activities at the Hospital de Base do Distrito Federal (HBDF), one of the largest and best-known public hospitals in the region. For this reason and because she is a librarian, she was invited to write an article about the work, in the form of an experience report, to be presented at the 27th Brazilian Congress of Librarianship and Documentation in 2017, a biannual event, whose theme was United Nations Sustainable Development Goals: how libraries can contribute to the implementation of the 2030 Agenda.

> The 2030 Agenda is an action plan for people, planet and prosperity, drawn up in September 2015 by representatives of the 193 UN Member States at a meeting in New York, where they recognised that the eradication of poverty in all its forms and dimensions, including extreme poverty, is the greatest global challenge and an indispensable requirement for sustainable development. The plan, which seeks to strengthen universal peace, indicates 17 Sustainable Development Goals (SDGs) and 169 targets to eradicate poverty and promote a decent life for all, within the limits of the planet. These are clear goals and targets for all countries to adopt according to their own priorities and act in the spirit of a global partnership that guides the choices needed to improve people's lives, now and in the future". (AGENDA 2030 PLATFORM).

The article, which gave rise to this book, was approved with maximum marks and priority for oral presentation, since its theme is aligned with two of the seventeen SDGs, namely: 3 - Ensure healthy lives and promote well-being for all at all ages; and 4 - Ensure inclusive and equitable quality education and promote lifelong learning opportunities for all. Thus, shortly after the congress, the approved articles were published in the proceedings of the event and, subsequently, the publisher Novas Edições Acadêmicas invited the author to write this book.

In her research, the author found bibliography that presents pilot and case studies, produced by students and researchers, in a predetermined period. These analyses were made with both fixed

3

groups, both of bibliotherapy applicators and patients, which made it possible to collect *feedback* from patients and provided clear results about the effectiveness of the application of the practice. Thus, the research carried out contributed richly to the scientific basis of this work and serves as a theoretical support capable of assisting in the understanding of the experience reported and the knowledge that emerged from it.

Firstly, the view of the applicator of the bibliotherapeutic technique and how he/she is affected by the process will be highlighted. In addition, it will be shown how bibliotherapy can be practised effectively in each type of public and different environments. All of this is based on a continuous experience of years of practice in the same hospital, with careful observation, constant learning, training, studies and research for improvement, as well as some random and spontaneous *feedback* from patients (testimonials, expressions of appreciation, applause, smiles, gestures of gratitude) and health professionals (with words of encouragement and support). At the end, there are testimonials from some of the bibliotherapy practitioners, who are volunteers of the Storytellers Group, to illustrate, with sincere words, everything that comprises the scope of these pages.

Thus, in order to enable more people to benefit, the author brings techniques, recommendations and suggestions related to bibliotherapy, both to the hospital and home environment. After sharing acquired knowledge, coordinated based on a set of practical experiences, which means the author's own personal transformation, a model of application of the art of storytelling will be presented, totally replicable by anyone interested in exercising this beautiful activity. And to bring more vividness to this research, in the chapter *Stories lived in the hospital*: endless lessons, there are true accounts in which the power of this practice can be demonstrated more eloquently.

Introduction

In all the traditions and cultures that exist on Earth, it is possible to observe the presence of stories in the development of civilisations. Created, told, metaphorical, true or fictional, they tell about life, customs, illusions, desires, dreams, ways of thinking, among others through which human beings recognise themselves as individuals and, above all, see themselves as social actors. In stories, we identify with the characters, we see in them qualities that we admire or would like to have and defects that we want or need to correct in ourselves. Often, we just observe and judge their way of being, supporting or not their attitudes, and this also teaches us to know who we are or who we want to be in the world.

In this way, stories have the great power to provide pleasant, interesting, relaxed moments and, at the same time, lead to an awakening to new possibilities, opportunities and conditions, previously unimaginable. Seen from this angle, narratives represent a great opportunity for self-knowledge, to look inside oneself and realise that this character, who lives there, also lives inside each one, but "asleep" or anaesthetised by events. Involved by thoughts and feelings, this protagonist is prevented from absorbing the best of experiences, so it is so necessary to awaken to their own potential, to act in favour of their evolution and, with that, discover the wonder that life can be.

The simple act of telling a story to someone, either by reading or by speaking, makes us realise how it is possible to be effective without being boring. In this sense, narrating shows us how to pass on a message, a positive message, a reflection or even a new idea, achieving high-value results, in a way that is not only pleasant, but also very effective. Its benefits are notorious in the professional, social, family, sports and, above all, health areas, which is the focus of this book.

Research around the world has revealed how *storytelling*, also known as *storytelling,* affects people much more powerfully, as it brings a lot of meaning to what you want to draw attention to. Through the studies, it was discovered that this method is more effective in getting a message across, as it engages people more emotionally, with less emphasis on the rational. And it was also realised that explaining theories and making elaborations can easily be replaced by a simple and well-told narration, as long as it brings a lot of relevance to the life of those who listen to it. In this way, it promotes a commotion of feelings that make the person more receptive and open to new information, because there is a much greater identification between sender and receiver, which generates empathy and, therefore, facilitates the promotion of ideas and products.

The practice of telling and listening to stories plays many roles in the formation and evolution of mankind and is seen as something very pleasurable and therapeutic. Stories of oral tradition, folklore, sacred, literary, biblical, or parables and fables, and also the stories of the theatre, cinema and soap opera, in short, whatever the origin or modality, all have their value, and provide more grace to live, being inexhaustible sources of teachings. Stories are responsible for shaping our conscience, behaviour, attitudes, customs and thus opening our hearts and minds to more possibilities.

Therefore, through bibliotherapy, it will be demonstrated how it is possible to realise the idea of therapeutic exchange provided by the use of books and narratives as instruments that give rise to an experience in which everyone benefits, since the act of storytelling symbolises a medicine for all, whose active principle is love.

CHAPTER 1

Storytelling Group: origin and evolution

> "Do what you can, with what you have, where you are."
>
> -- Theodore Roosevelt

In 2011, an activity that put into practice the concepts of bibliotherapy was initiated in a public hospital in Brasília (DF), even though at the time there was no technical knowledge on the subject, the first step was taken to create the Storytellers group. A member of the Spiritist Communion of Brasilia (CEB) had this idea and, with the Department of Social Promotion of this institution, presented the work proposal to the Base Hospital of the Federal District, which was approved The group was linked at the time to the Voluntary Auxiliary Service (SAV). It then began its work with only four volunteers.

As the work was widely publicised and new coordinators joined, many people became interested in learning about the initiative and taking part. Thus, there was an expansion with the entry of people of different ages, professions, beliefs, etc., and to join, the only prerequisites were the age of majority (or being over fourteen accompanied/authorised by a guardian) and good will.

The group started working at the Hospital de Base do Distrito Federal in the first half of 2011 on Thursdays from 2.30pm to 5pm, with stories only for children. Then more people became interested in working on Wednesdays, and later on Saturdays. Thus, three teams were formed: Wednesday, Thursday and Saturday, each with their own coordinators, but volunteers were free to work on any of the three days or even on more than one.

In the beginning, the group was linked to the Voluntary Auxiliary Service of the HBDF, one of the associations that has a room in the hospital, with volunteers, who took turns to keep it open during the week. Donations of material for the patients were received there, and a bazaar was kept for the sale of clothes and new items. The funds raised were used to buy material for the patients.

The Voluntary Auxiliary Service organised teams of volunteers who offer a range of services to patients. After five years, we were redirected and became linked to the Associação Amigos do Hospital de Base, another organisation that also brings together teams of volunteers and has a room in the hospital with similar characteristics to the previous one.

The Associação Amigos do Hospital de Base (AAHB), to which the group is currently linked, provides all the administrative procedures related to the access and circulation of volunteers in the establishment. In the room where the AAHB operates, all the group's work material, such as books and folders with stories, is kept. It is also the place where the volunteers meet and prepare before going up to the wards to actually begin this beautiful, loving and therapeutic exchange of storytelling.

6

At the end, they also gather to store the material used and exchange information and reflections.

Over the years, the work has grown a lot, and with its repercussion came the invitation to also implement the activity at the Armed Forces Hospital (HFA) in 2015. At first, a small team was formed that worked in the afternoon, in the medical clinic area, which later expanded to the morning, in the emergency room. In this hospital, the group was linked to the Friends of the HFA Association (ASAHFA), but with stricter rules for volunteering, so the team was fixed.

How to become a volunteer storyteller? To join the Storytellers group, you need to contact the team and make an appointment with one of the coordinators, on one of the days that the work takes place. The suggestion is always for the candidate to accompany the activity for a day to get to know the work. Only after that, he decides if he will continue. Choosing to continue, this new volunteer will be on trial for about a month (to see if he will really adapt). After this period, he/she will be interviewed by the AAHB secretary, who will arrange for registration and an identification badge. The group also provides a lilac lab coat on permanent loan, which must be worn on the hospital premises while working.

At the HFA, the group's activities take place at fixed locations on Tuesdays (morning and afternoon) and consist of telling stories to patients, military personnel of the armed forces or their dependents, who are hospitalised or those in the emergency room.

At Hospital de Base, the tasks take place on Wednesday, Thursday and Saturday afternoons. The public served is very varied, made up of people in more vulnerable social conditions, from the Federal District and other states of Brazil. The volunteers divide into small groups and distribute themselves on the floors planned for that day. In total, there are eleven floors, each with approximately twelve rooms, each with two or four beds.

On the day of the work, the volunteers gather in the AAHB or ASAHFA room, sign the attendance list, read the story of the day and end with a brief reflection. Those who go to the paediatric ward gather the books to take away and prepare with props, puppets, etc. The others go up to the programmed floors with copies of the stories - some also use props. There is a voice preparation with some quick exercises. And sometimes, on the way, a prayer is said before and after the activity.

In adult wards, some motivational stories are told. Volunteers enter the rooms in pairs or groups of three or four people, introduce themselves, greet those present, distribute the copies and perform the storytelling. Afterwards, they stimulate a conversation about the narration, which usually serves as an opening for reflections, outbursts, life stories, etc. There is a good participation, but some participants do not speak due to their illness. In some situations, the stories are left at the bedside for the patient or carer to read when they return to consciousness. Often, at the end, games are played such as riddles, charades, jokes, and the patients have a lot of fun trying to answer them. This creates an atmosphere of relaxation and good humour among the patients and the group.

On the 11th floor of the Hospital de Base, there is a ward called Papudinha. This is where patients, male or female, who need hospital treatment but are serving time in the Papuda Penitentiary Complex in the Federal District are kept. They are handcuffed to stretchers. This sector is separated by a grid, with a security system, and is heavily guarded by prison officers who remain on site daily controlling everything that comes in and out of there. The volunteers of the Storytellers Group are generally authorised to enter and tell the story of the day to the inmates, provided they follow some security guidelines.

With children it is quite different. The children's audience is made up of children and adolescents between 0 and 18 years old. The 7th floor of the Hospital de Base, where the paediatrics department is located, is decorated in a playful way and has a room called Escolinha, where two teachers are located. In this room, the group always tells stories to those present and has the full support of the teachers. In addition, patients do their schoolwork and have at their disposal books, educational games, puzzles, drawing and colouring material, as well as the help of educators for their activities. It is worth mentioning that children's books are used throughout the paediatric ward.

Considering the diversity of the children's audience, volunteers use other resources to attract attention to the books and make the moment more fun, such as songs and nursery rhymes for babies, magic, puppets and riddles for teenagers. In addition, a few extra copies of the day's story are taken for the carers to tell the stories to sleeping children.

It is essential to highlight that all the work of the volunteers, as soon as they arrive on each floor, is preceded by hand hygiene, with guidance from the nursing staff on possible restrictions of contamination. This procedure occurs for the mutual safety and protection of patients and volunteers, and also serves to ensure that the employees of the floor served are always aware of the presence of the group that day.

The general coordination is of great relevance, as it is responsible for the financial part of the group, which includes intermediation with the institution that provides this financial support for making lab coats and printing copies of the stories. It is also responsible for selecting, editing and printing the narratives that will be taken to the hospital for distribution and reading. The general coordination also informs weekly, through the group formed in the WhatsApp application, the programme of floors for each day of work, so that there are no repetitions in the week, since a single story is used for all floors.

It should also be noted that the representatives of the group attend annual accountability meetings at the Hospital de Base. All volunteer associations are called to participate so that the results of their activities can be taken to the Public Prosecutor's Office. This practice supports the work of volunteers at the hospital, in addition to providing an annual report of activities to the institution that sponsors the group with the work material.

Hospital staff always show full support for the group's activities, not only by providing necessary information, but also by including the group in the hospital's programme. Doctors, nurses, physiotherapists, psychologists, speech therapists, assistants, teachers, kitchen staff and cleaning staff know about the group and understand the relevance of the work for the improvement and well-being of patients. A good example of this is the fact that a speech therapist from Hospital de Base has already given free training to volunteers at a training *workshop* organised by the group's coordinators.

Throughout these years, the group has undergone many changes and has evolved a lot. Several meetings have been held between the coordinators to make decisions, resolve issues, better organise the group's activities or create necessary rules, in addition to the training courses that have been given to volunteers. In addition, in 2015, a seminar was held at the Federal Senate entitled Early Childhood and Epigenetics, in which the group participated and gave a workshop. On that occasion, the knowledge acquired by the group in these years of experience was shared, and the most experienced storytellers shared their knowledge.

In 2018, the Storytelling Group - DPS has about ninety volunteers. The experience acquired over all these years allows us to affirm that the work carried out contributes to a more humanised hospitalisation, fills the usual idleness of patients with pleasant moments of relaxation, learning, joy and leisure, in addition to effectively collaborating in a therapeutic way in the lives of patients, companions and volunteers.

Hospital de Base do Distrito Federal

It is known that it was created within the guidelines of a new health system for the new capital, called the Bandeira de Mello Plan. In addition to a bold architectural structure, the aim was to offer public services to the new population of the capital, with a focus on preventive rather than curative care, and collective rather than individual assistance. The implementation of this plan culminated in the creation of a management body called the DF Hospital Foundation (FHDF). The Base Hospital was created at the centre of the system. The aim was to offer modern public services, not only in relation to other regions of the country, but also to the world. The HBDF was built to be a highly complex centre. Around it were eleven general hospitals and six rural hospitals, a network of basic services capable of providing care for a population of 500,000 by the year 2000. From the 1970s onwards, this plan had to be revised (R. MÉDICO EM DIA, June 2017, p. 23).

This institution that was born to have excellence in high complexity health services and also in teaching and research, over all these years of existence, has become an intangible heritage of the DF, such is its importance and representativeness.

The hospital has approximately 5,000 employees daily: 3,700 staff (doctors, nurses, health technicians, administrators); 400 resident doctors, excluding outsourced workers (cleaning, security, assistants); and serves thousands of patients daily. In view of the increase in population and administrative and financial difficulties, in 2017 the hospital was transformed into an institute, having been renamed Instituto Hospital de Base do DF (IHBDF).

The structure of the IHBDF is composed of several buildings, divided into sectors, which practically form a hospital complex. In its tallest building, with eleven floors, are the wards, where the Storytelling Group - DPS carries out its activities. The specialities that operate on each floor are:

2. Orthopaedics
3. Neurosurgery
4. Cardiology/Thoracic Surgery
5. Angiology/Gynaecology/Bucomaxillary
6. General surgery
7. Paediatrics
8. Neurology and Urology
9. Nephrology (dialysis, haemodialysis, kidney transplantation)
10. Oncology (endocrinology, pulmonology)
11. Medical practice and infectology (rheumatology, gastroenterology) - Papudinha

There are also many volunteer associations at the Instituto Hospital de Base, in addition to the Associação Amigos do Hospital de Base (Friends of the Base Hospital Association), such as the SAV (Auxiliary Volunteer Service), the Movimento de Apoio ao Paciente com Câncer (MAC) (Cancer Patient Support Movement) and the Rede Feminina de Combate ao Câncer (Women's Network to Fight Cancer). Within them there are specific groups, such as: Reiki application in patients; beauty (which provides hair cutting and painting services, manicure and pedicure in patients); Anjalhaços (which plays games); and bed support (which provides free hygiene and personal use materials to patients who cannot afford them). It is worth noting that the largest group of volunteers at the hospital, with about eighty registered members, is the Storytellers Group.

CHAPTER 2

Bibliotherapy: a different focus

"Love without expecting to be loved, and without expecting any reward."
(Chico Xavier)

Much of the literature on bibliotherapy brings the approach of "supportive reading" with therapeutic potential and can also be seen as reading mediation work, i.e. the approach given to the process is that a person, or a group, works to help physically or mentally disadvantaged patients by applying therapeutic reading followed by a dialogue with these sick or vulnerable individuals who, passively or actively, receive the wonderful effects of bibliotherapy.

According to Seitz (2006), the term bibliotherapy is derived from the Greek *biblion*, which designates all types of bibliographic or reading material, and *therapein*, which means treatment, cure or restoration. Rubin (apud VASQUEZ, 1989, p. 22) defines the concept as "a programme of activities based on the interactive process of the people who experience it. The material, printed or not, imaginative or informative, is experienced and discussed with the help of a facilitator". For Buonocori (apud ALVES, 1982, p. 55), bibliotherapy "is the art of curing illness through reading".

In the international scientific literature, it can be seen that the subject has numerous research and case studies around the world. Universities have specific departments, faculties and postgraduate programmes to study the subject. Historically, it is known that the use of reading for therapeutic purposes has been practised for centuries. In ancient Egypt, Pharaoh Ramesses II wrote at the entrance to his library: "Remedies for the soul". In contemporary cinema, in the film *The Girl Who Stole Books*, which takes place during the World War, the main character reads to a sick cousin who is staying at his house, he says that reading played a fundamental role in restoring his health.

For Caldin (2010), who had his research guided by a pilot study in a hospital, it can be said that bibliotherapy is the possibility of therapy through literary texts, since it is not only configured as a reading (narration or dramatisation), but also because it contemplates the comments arising from what is read, born of the listener's experiences, and merges with the interpretation of the author's words. And he adds that bibliotherapy is not limited to reading, narrating and dramatising a text, since it goes further by prioritising listening to the new text arising from the creation of each of those involved in the reading session. In other words, it means exchanging experiences without losing sight of the individualisation of the subject. Bibliotherapy, therefore, is defined as a cyclical process in which the act of reading or telling stories with subsequent dialogue, if possible, is seen as a moment or experience that provides therapeutic benefits to those involved in the activity.

11

In this process, the participating subjects - storytellers or listeners - are seen as human beings in their complexities, and therefore both are analysed for the effects of bibliotherapy. For the convalescent, the dynamics of listening to the story, interpreting it and talking about it or not is considered therapeutic, because of the various beneficial effects caused, which will be discussed later. For those who tell or read the story and then talk about it, a series of positive effects can also be identified.

For Castro and Pinheiro (2005, p. 3), bibliotherapy is "an interactive process of feelings, values and actions, resulting in a harmonious and balanced process of personal growth and development". This undoubtedly occurs at various levels for each of those involved in the dynamic.

In this sense, another important piece of information is that the practice of bibliotherapy should be preceded by the joint reading of the story(s) to be used and by dialogue on its various interpretations by its applicators. This moment of union and sharing is already extremely therapeutic and prepares the applicator, both emotionally, by allowing him to feel and appease the feelings aroused by the text, and technically, by providing a repertoire of interpretations that foster more fruitful debates with patients. Thus, the benefit of bibliotherapy begins with the applicator, who becomes able to deal with the various situations that may occur during the practice.

However, there is no way of judging who needs some kind of therapy more, who is better or worse off in terms of physical or mental health. This is why the whole process is considered a therapeutic exchange, not least because the roles of the actors are sometimes reversed. Thus everyone is perceived with a certain level of equality.

The following questions will help you better understand what has been said.

- Can't the wounds of the (hidden) soul be greater or more painful than those of the physical body?
- Isn't the person telling a story also listening to it?
- Can't those who tell stories also listen to many others?

The patient goes to hospital seeking to improve their physical or mental condition and inevitably experiences a breakdown of physical and emotional patterns. This is mainly due to the abandonment of their normal routine to stay for a period of time in hospital. Thus, he is forced to live in a different environment, with different people and habits, in addition to a series of limitations that force him to change, however little, his way of seeing life.

That is why bibliotherapy is perceived as an equitable action among those involved. It should be emphasised that, from the patients' point of view, pure hospitalisation already promotes a certain rupture of patterns, which facilitates a change of consciousness and attitudes. Although the patients are in apparently more limited health conditions, most of them are more open to stories, more flexible and prone to dialogues and reflections. From the storyteller's perspective, the storyteller experiences a rupture of patterns of consciousness when listening to the life narratives of the sick, which are full of lessons. With this, he also receives his extra doses of therapy.

Human contact through the telling of a story, eye to eye, in which permission is asked to start a conversation through a story or a book, brings warmth, affection, attention to people often lacking all this. And through this door, a path opens to beautiful perceptions for all participants in this activity, about their own conditions, possibilities, self-knowledge, always with a common goal that flows into self-love and love for others.

Telling and listening to stories helps us to build ourselves as people, to understand ourselves, to see ourselves in the world, as well as transporting us to other universes and bringing us other senses. It frees us from insistent thoughts, gives us a break from the problems that afflict us and teaches us other ways of seeing the world, other realities. In addition, it leads us to reflect on our lives and shows us simplified and even very funny ways of looking at life. This experience makes us stop, listen, interpret, dialogue and, with this, see how much, at the same time, it empties us of what we should leave behind and fills us with new feelings, new emotions, just because someone cares, someone tells a story with all the affection and is there to listen carefully, someone wants to hear your "voice" or simply let the story itself stay there resonating in the silence of your heart.

CHAPTER 3

10 "commandments" of storytellers working in hospitals

"Strength does not come from physical ability. It comes from an indomitable will."
(Mahatma Gandhi)

The list of guidelines listed below, in the form of ten commandments, was drawn up in 2012 for the Storytellers Group (DPS). The accelerated growth of the group, due to the arrival of new volunteers interested in experiencing bibliotherapy, made it necessary to put on paper some basic guidelines that are essential, allowing easy and quick reading. At that time and over the years, a number of other documents were produced, such as manuals, reports, training material and lectures.

However, the guidelines only fulfil the purpose of providing information in a summarised and easy-to-understand way, so that people without any experience or training can start this activity accompanied by more experienced bibliotherapy practitioners. In this way, as a participant for a day, a lay person can get to know how it works and, after that, decide if they really want to incorporate this activity as a weekly commitment, for example, in their life. These guidelines can be used and applied in any bibliotherapy group working in a hospital.

The 10 commandments of the Storyteller who works in hospital:

1. You'll always keep a smile on your face while working, bringing joy and positivity to those you meet at the hospital.

2. You will identify yourself and greet everyone in the room.

3. You will maintain proper hygiene when entering and leaving the rooms.

4. You will not ask patients about their illness or treatment.

5. You will tell stories appropriate to the age groups they are aimed at.

6. You will keep your work materials and handle them with care.

7. You will listen carefully to patients and carers, as letting off steam may do them good.

8. You will try to understand the times when it is better to let them rest or be alone with their relatives/friends.

9. You will always tell positive, reflective and humorous stories.

10. You will not carry out activities that fall outside the remit of a storyteller.

CHAPTER 4

The art of telling and listening to stories!

"Pills relieve pain, but only love relieves suffering".

(Author unknown)

Storytelling for therapeutic purposes requires something inexplicably indispensable: a deep sense of love. It is important to clarify that it is the love transmitted through the activity that makes it therapeutic. This feeling contains empathy, compassion, humility, attention, in short, all the attributes necessary to provide listening, understanding, dialogue or the (sometimes necessary) silence that follows after the story. This love is felt by those who participate in the bibliotherapeutic activity.

For this reason, the application of the practice in the domestic environment, from mother to child, from father to child, from grandmother to grandchild, from grandchild to grandparent, is highly recommended, since love, in general, is a feeling that already permeates these relationships. In addition, the listener's profile and literary taste are better known, which facilitates the choice of stories to be applied and makes possible a more personalised and perhaps even more effective bibliotherapy.

So who can apply the technique? Everyone, it is enough that the activity is carried out as a way of transmitting love. The only caveat regarding the application of the practice in hospital environments is the formation of a group or team so that the work is done in an organised manner and in accordance with the hospital's rules.

Do you have to be in health care, hospitalised or convalescent to receive bibliotherapy? Of course not, it acts even on those who think they are less needy, especially on the one who tells the story! Just as it also acts on plants, animals and everything around, because the wave of love carried through the intention of the storyteller, and through the story itself, resonates wherever it goes without distinction.

In the hospital environment, bibliotherapy practitioners deal with hospitalised patients and their companions, i.e. completely unknown people, without any emotional bond. However, it is very impressive to realise how effective and profound the practice is despite this ignorance. Thus, as unusual as it may seem, this feeling exists, since otherwise the experience would not be effective.

How are people able to transmit love to others they don't know? How is this feeling activated? When telling stories to a stranger, keeping in mind that your role there is to bring the best you can through a story, with the aim of providing a moment of relief and distraction in the period of pain and

16

suffering of that human being, it is obvious that love is intrinsic from the first intention and that there is no bibliotherapy without it. And the most incredible thing is that the transforming power of this feeling, which begins with an intention and manifests itself in an action, resonates mainly in those who are transmitting it, through cures, learning and unimaginable experiences, which represents the bibliotherapeutic magic.

On the other hand, sometimes the storyteller/listener himself enjoys the story, the conversation, feels the well-being provided by the moment and moves into a much more positive, good-humoured, confident and high-spirited state, but does not perceive very clearly more concrete results in his health. The reason is that in some cases this is only realised some time later, because of the naturalness and subtlety of bibliotherapy. In this case, one realises that the action of the practice works like a loving seed that is planted, but its flowers only appear later.

According to studies and observations, we know that it is practically impossible to separate body and mind, and for those who are storytellers it is very clear how one acts on the other. Therefore, it is understood that this more positive, good-humoured and confident state, provided by bibliotherapy, generates direct reflexes in the physical body. As a result, it is concluded that every gain in physical health reflects positively on emotional health, and vice versa.

In this way,

> [...] the close connection between illness and emotions could not go unmentioned, since the human being is one. It is known that intense emotions cause, in addition to failures in the immune system, real suffering and that it, even without defined organic causes, deserves care. It is not the case to say that every disease has its origin in feelings, but to verify how to minimise, by reading, the harmful effects of psychophysical problems, because the mismatch between body and mind breaks the harmony necessary for well-being. (CALDIN, 2010, p. 19).

In this sense, it is interesting to emphasise that some of the beliefs that the storytellers had in relation to this mind-body interaction were dissolving over the years of practice. The main one was that they had to be very well physically and emotionally to practice bibliotherapy in the hospital. They believed it was indispensable to be extremely psychologically balanced to deal with all the harshness of the scenes witnessed in the hospital environment. Likewise, they thought it was important to be physically well for this activity, when, in fact, the only restriction for the performance of a storyteller is to carry some contagious disease, in order to avoid the risk of infecting patients.

Thus, after a few lessons and experiences, bibliotherapy practitioners today do not hesitate to put their hands to work, even if they are in some physical or emotional discomfort. This is due to the clear realisation that they are also directly and positively affected by the activity, which is why they have found in practice that the pains they may have felt at the end of the day have diminished or ended. What about emotional discomfort? This is what first disappears, giving way to joy, contentment, gratitude, in other words, generating a feeling of internal fulfilment, as if life gained more meaning. This is the phenomenon of the double action of bibliotherapy.

Thus, those who do not imagine how the phenomenon happens believe that they will find it very difficult to convey love to unknown people. There is only one thing to say: start! Apply bibliotherapy just once! And you will see that your sincere intention, together with this fabulous attitude, will move formidable energies and when you least expect it you will be naturally experiencing this fantastic experience of love in the form of stories.

Here are some explanations for this phenomenon of the double action of bibliotherapy.

1. **Congruence in action**: since bibliotherapy practitioners believe that those who participate in listening and talking about stories improve their health, then those who tell, listen and talk about the story, several times in one day and experiencing every aspect of this experience, are sure of the effectiveness of the action and that they are also affected by this process, this is congruence.

> Conventional medicine already recognises that common experience can play a complex role in disease. For example, statistics show that singles and widowers are more susceptible to cancer than married people. Their loneliness is called a risk factor (CHOPRA, 2015, p. 32).

2. **Shift of focus**: bibliotherapy practitioners take the focus off their own pain and what ails them to give their best, in their most motivated, joyful and positive state, to be able to soothe the feelings of the people they come into contact with, in order to alleviate those delicate moments they are going through. This willingness triggers high vibrational frequency energies, represented by feelings of love, gratitude, joy, acceptance, etc.

According to renowned psychiatrist Dr David R. Hawkins, creator of the Table of Consciousness, everything you vibrate through feelings and emotions comes back to yourself. See the following Figure.

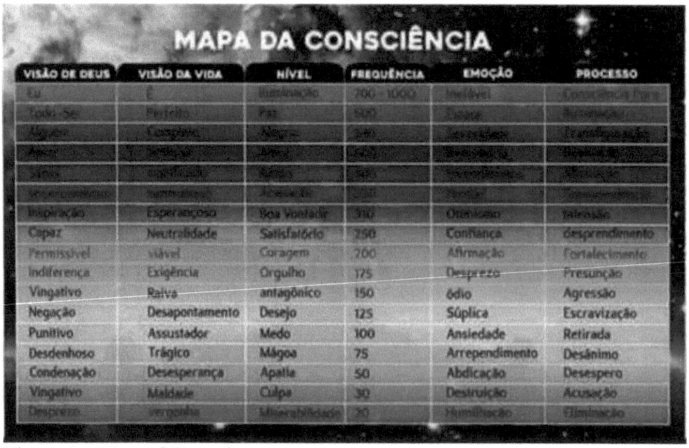

Figure 1 - Map of Consciousness

vibrate-can-be-measured-and-it-influences-your-destination/.
Accessed on: 9 Oct. 2018.

3. **Change of consciousness**: the situations that bibliotherapy applicators witness in the hospital environment transform them profoundly. Each day of stories represents a learning experience that makes them see other perspectives of their own lives. In addition, the interaction with patients and caregivers, through their stories, outbursts, attitudes and behaviours, teaches the storytellers a lot about life. This makes them expand their consciousness and broaden their view of everything in the universe. Thus, the participants start to value their own health much more, everything becomes simpler and more uncomplicated, problems become easier to deal with. small.

CHAPTER 5

Recommendations and techniques

> "It is not our talents that show us who we really are, but our
> choices."
>
> (film *Harry Potter and the Secret Chamber*)

Some recommendations are necessary regarding the application of bibliotherapy. This is due to the care that must be taken in contact with the sick and with all those who are present in the same environment in which one or more stories are told for therapeutic purposes. These places, whether domestic or hospital, must be respected so that bibliotherapy really achieves its purpose and works as an aid in the treatment or recovery of the individual.

Thus, the moment of application of the bibliotherapeutic technique with adults begins with the narration of the story and has objectives aimed at reflection and dialogue on the themes addressed, the message that the story passes, the interpretations employed and also the participants' own life stories. Many take the opportunity to vent difficulties or situations that occurred in the past that are rescued by the text. For these reasons, it appears that for adults bibliotherapy represents a form of welcome, attention, love, affection and sensitivity, which contributes to raising their self-esteem, self-confidence, their good humour, in addition to easing stress and relieving worry and anxiety generated by treatment or recovery period.

On the other hand, the application of this practice in children has a much more playful bias, directed to awaken them to reading as something positive and pleasurable. They are involved through imagination, fun and joy, without much focus on reflections.

Techniques for the application of Bibliotherapy

1. **Knowledge of stories**:

   Adults: research good stories that are suitable for the style you want, read and study it beforehand, feel the emotions it provokes, dig deep into the message it conveys, talk to colleagues about the different interpretations it can have, the hooks it can provide to carry motivating and empowering messages.

   Children: get to know children's books well enough to choose the most appropriate one according to the child's age and moment. It is worth noting that some children's books also arouse interest in adults, because the magic provided by these stories that escape reality help them to have a moment of pause in the hard routine of treatment or the factual situation in which they find themselves. In addition, many of these narratives are metaphors created by adults and adapted to children's vocabulary.

2. **Diction and speech:** warm up your voice with exercises taught by a speech therapist to loosen your tongue, improve your diction and speak clearly, at a speed and volume adapted to each situation.

3. **Forming pairs and congruent groups:** always work in groups of at least two volunteers in a hospital environment, so that they develop a harmonious and sensitive performance. There is no recommendation for this in the home environment.

4. **Creating closeness:** always start the contact by greeting the people present and introducing yourself. Then ask or read the name of the patient(s) and call them by name, both during the storytelling and in the subsequent dialogue.

5. **Checking the willingness of potential listeners:** asking if people want to hear stories.

   <u>Adults:</u> in general, the answer is yes. However, when it comes to several people, such as in a hospital room, some accept and others do not. In this case, the situation of the moment is evaluated and the decision is made, which is usually to tell the story. When this happens, at the end, you can see the satisfaction generated in everyone present, including those who refused.

   <u>Children:</u> some children in treatment sleep or are in fragile situations. Therefore, it is very common for them not to want to listen to stories at that time, which must be fully respected by the storyteller. Others say they do not like books or stories, or even say they do not want to because they are irritated at that moment. Many of them have never heard a story, so they are not able to judge whether they like it or not. It also happens that they have heard a narration in a way that they did not like. And it is at this moment that we have the opportunity to change this negative pattern of the past and to create a new look at what stories are and what they are capable of providing to listeners.

   Some alternatives for these cases are:

   1. Tell the story to other children who are around, (at the end it is possible that you are visibly participating or enjoying the storytelling).

   2. Tell the child that he/she is going through a test. Tell them that you are going to tell the story just to let them know if they can tell it well or badly, if they agree, start the storytelling.

   3. Make some guesses (Chapter 6) at first to provoke an opening to the story, a change of mood in the child, then start telling if you realise that the strategy has worked.

6. **Joy and good humour**: being in a happy and positive mood is essential for bibliotherapy to achieve good results, since the goal is also to change the mood of the room and make people more motivated and optimistic. Thus, it is recommended to use colourful and fun props to promote a pattern break. This practice, because it is unexpected, has a positive influence. It relaxes, amuses, is irreverent and puts people in a more receptive state.

7. **Division of the story**: it is interesting that the bibliotherapy providers, if there is more than one, alternate in the narration of the paragraphs of the story to give dynamism and distribute the activity evenly. In the case of children, the storytellers can change the lines in the parts of the book or take over the speech of the characters, changing the voice, playing games, using puppets or singing children's songs in the middle of the story.

8. **Sensitivity and intuition:** talking, listening and silence, in each case an option. After the story, for the adults, give rise to a constructive dialogue, asking them what they thought, if they liked it, if the story has any message for them, etc.

9. **Know how to listen:** If there are spontaneous comments, listen and encourage the venting. During this conversation, volunteers should never use a moralising tone, ask about the history that creates embarrassment or invade the individuality of patients.

10. **Charades moment**: we recommend at the end to use a technique to bring a little more relaxation and lightness to the enclosure, whenever possible, which consists of making some riddles, charades, jokes or funny things for everyone to have fun. We have realised that this is very effective for both children and adults. After all, as the saying goes "laughter is the best medicine".

The lessons received each day as a storyteller provide much healing, growth and maturation to those who decide to dedicate themselves, even once a week, to this type of practice, especially those who manage to act with true awareness, not only telling, but also listening and vigorously absorbing the countless messages that a single story carries, even children's stories. Even more so to those who have the sensitivity to really listen to what the sick tell them about themselves and realise that true wisdom comes through unexpected paths, you just have to be open to receive it.

Techniques to bring stories to life

Putting life into the story makes all the difference!

A narrative can be told in many ways. Regardless of who tells it, their way of being, preferences, etc., the fact of telling a story to someone is already a very commendable act that, in itself, can already be considered extremely relevant on certain occasions. However, knowing the therapeutic reach of this wonderful gesture, we draw attention to techniques that may be able to improve the quality of this experience, making it much more attractive and effective in its purpose.

Making the voices of the characters, putting sound effects, onomatopoeia, singing a song, when appropriate, dialogue, bringing the child into the story, to be part of the world of the characters, is something that transforms a simple story into a magical moment, which will be eternalized in the memory of that little human being, who will grow up with a healthier, more creative mind, believing more in life, in their abilities, in addition to realizing that reading can be very fun and enjoyable.

Recommendations: bibliotherapy for adults

In order to enjoy this time in the best possible way, the following precautions are important:

1 Conscious choice of story

Select motivating and positive stories that carry empowering messages and fulfil the therapeutic purpose.

2 Rhythm and emotion

Tell the story with emotion and rhythm, if possible looking into the eyes of the listeners, at least in some moments, providing dynamism and fluidity to the text.

3 Meaning *versus* interpretation

Always observe the meaning of the story so that misinterpretations of the text are avoided, leading to conflict of ideas when there is more than one listener. If there is any discrepancy in interpretation, lead to a positive conclusion, one of love and understanding.

4 Adaptation of the text

If there are foreign names of characters, ambiguous words that may generate a double meaning, discomfort or negative interpretation of the text, change these names to others that are more harmonised with local customs.

Recommendations: bibliotherapy for children

1 Profile observation

It is essential to choose a book according to the profile and age group of the children. This requires careful observation of the storyteller and a brief conversation with the children or their carers. We have already told stories to Indian patients, foreigners or patients from other distant states, with very different languages, customs or ways of life, not to mention socioeconomic variations. Therefore, it is essential to pay attention to these factors when choosing a story, as it is always preferable that the child can identify and understand what is being told as much as possible. This way, they will really have fun and enjoy the moment in the most beneficial way.

2 Unheard/Repeated Always ask if the child has heard that story before to avoid repetition, unless the child asks to hear it again.

3 Being an actor/actress

Telling the story, more than simply reading the text, really interpreting it, entering the narration, the world of the characters.

4 Dialogues

Promote dialogues between the book/characters and the child patient, when possible, bringing them into the story as an active participant.

5 Unforeseen/Improvised

Improvise with the text of the book when necessary to adapt it to the situation of the moment, or situations that arise during the telling of the story, being able to abbreviate, speed up or cut parts of a story, for example.

*Patients may experience a variety of situations when telling a story, from the approach of people who draw their attention, taking the focus away from the story, to complications related to the physical state of the patient, so the flexibility of the storyteller is necessary to adapt to each case.

6 Images/Illustrations

Showing the pictures and illustrations of the book to the children who are listening to the story is more fun, dynamic and helps them understand and interpret what is being read.

7 Puppets

Use puppets to talk to the children about the story or to be the characters if appropriate.

8 Music

Sing some music/song related to the book/characters if you feel it is appropriate. In the case of babies, this is usually desirable.

9 Freedom of speech

Allow the child to make comments about the story or the characters, even if it interrupts the story.

CHAPTER 6

Approaching hospitalised patients: feeling before speaking

"We all have something to heal at some level of our being."

(Fabyola Lima Madeira)

Sensing the atmosphere of the environment is fundamental to beginning a patient approach. The guideline is to always enter each ward room with your senses alert. Being present, with full awareness at that moment, is the key to acting as a good observer. Based on this, find the best way to initiate the approach and start the bibliotherapeutic process.

In this chapter, some guidelines and perceptions will be exposed, coming more specifically from the experience as a participant in the Storytellers Group, which operates at the Base Hospital of the Federal District. Therefore, it is information based on the practice of bibliotherapy within the hospital environment.

At the Hospital de Base, each week, the group's teams are always taking turns on the floors. Therefore, it is possible to meet a diversity of people (babies, children, adolescents, adults, elderly) and situations. Examples include patients:
- in advanced stages of disease.
- with chronic illnesses who spend periods in hospital, and we always meet them again.
- awaiting surgery.
- who are convalescing from surgery.
- in long treatments.
- who have suffered accidents, in recovery.
- with neurological problems.
- in a coma.
- who have lost their memory.

The socio-economic situation of the people treated in a public hospital is very varied. There has been contact with homeless patients, indigenous people, others from cities in the interior of Bahia, Maranhão, Goiás, who came by ambulance and even foreigners who did not speak fluent Portuguese. We also identified that many people bring sheets, blankets, towels and personal supplies from home

25

to the hospital. However, others do not have any of this, they only use what the space provides or what the hospital's volunteer teams donate, such as personal hygiene material. In short, the social status of the patients is predominantly low.

The inmate patients, who come from the DF prison system, are all on the 11th floor (which is the last floor of the infirmary building), regardless of gender, in a specific wing, which they call "Papudinha". It is a part separated by bars and protected by prison guards, who control the entry and exit of people and materials 24 hours a day. In addition, the prisoners are handcuffed to their beds during their hospitalisation. The volunteers of the Storytellers group are generally authorised to enter and tell the narrative to these patients, provided they follow some security guidelines. Their goodwill and receptivity to the story is always noticeable.

Some people question why they tell stories to prisoners, others say that the group should not serve them because they are criminals and therefore do not deserve to receive this "good deed". In fact, none of the hospital patients are known to the group members, nor is it even known what brought them there, even because there is a policy of not going into the merits of the illness/treatment. In addition, the role of those who practice bibliotherapy is not to judge anyone, but to bring a positive and motivating message through stories and dialogue, as this can reflect a better future for that human being, as well as great learning for the participants. Very wise words have already been spoken by them, despite the condition of being sentenced. Thus, we believe in the transformative power of bibliotherapy, and this is preponderant.

Another point to note, the chaperone is compulsory for children. For adults, it is optional. In the case of prisoners, the prison guard is the one who fulfils this role. Thus, there is a great variety on the part of these carers. Some go through the problem with more optimism, see the more serious cases around them and console themselves or even feel grateful that their loved one's situation is not so serious. Many, however, are extremely worn out and apparently overwhelmed by the hospital routine, the anxiety to get out of there soon and the lack of option to resume their activities, their work, family life, in short, their life.

Most of the rooms have four beds, where four patients stay with their respective carers. There are a few single or double rooms where more severe cases or those requiring isolation usually stay. All rooms have a bathroom and a television. It is noticeable that in the quadruple dormitories people make friends and help each other. They keep each other company, talk, share their anxieties. Despite the inconvenience of having to share a single bathroom, the discomfort that sometimes one wants silence and the other wants to watch television, these benefits are noted in the coexistence within the wards.

The visits take place at the same time as the work of the Storytelling Group. Thus, sometimes the participants enter a place full of visitors, when they are in that moment of missing each other, talking, when the patients feel loved and welcomed. There are no restrictions on this, as the stories have already been told in rooms full of visitors. In general, everyone welcomes the idea of taking a break to listen to a story, reflect or laugh a little. The emotional condition generated by the illness usually also affects family and friends who come to visit. We therefore believe that the story also has a positive effect on visitors.

Hospital procedures occur incessantly. Changing dressings or nappies, administering medication, delivering food, physiotherapy, psychological counselling etc. happen very often as we move from room to room. For this reason, the group follows some guidelines regarding the approach in order to carry out the work without affecting the harmony of the existing hospital processes.

Pre-approach guidelines:

- **At the bedroom door:** if the door is closed, knock lightly and open.
- **Assess the environment:** if it is open, look at the door and assess whether it is appropriate to enter at that time.
- **Come back later:** if any kind of medical procedure is taking place, such as dressing changes, tube, nappy, bed change, or if the patient is feeling unwell, do not enter the room and return later.
- **Do not enter:** in case of patient death or if there is a contamination hazard warning on the door.
- **Sanitisation:** before entering, sanitise hands with alcohol gel.

Guidance during the actual approach:

- **Greeting/presentation:** enter and move around environments where patients and/or companions/visitors are present always with joy and sensitivity to perceive the type of action and behaviour to be adopted:
  1 ask permission to enter;
  2 give a general greeting to everyone present: "good morning", "good afternoon";
  3 introduce yourself and the group;
  4 ask if the group can tell stories at that time and if those present want to listen;
  5 ask, if not, if they want to keep the story to read it later;
  6 greet each patient by name (which is written at the top of their beds). For children, take the opportunity to ask their age;
- **Voice volume:** start the storytelling by graduating the voice volume according to the patients' situation. If someone is asleep, lower the voice so as not to wake them.
- **Children:** depending on the age of the child(ren), they are asked to choose the desired book from the options that the storyteller finds interesting according to the observed profile.

27

- **Delivery of the story in silence:** if everyone is asleep, enter in silence and leave the story at the patient's bedside.
- **Never:** ask the patient, carer or visitor the reason for hospitalisation;
- **Never:** ask what the patient's carer is, whether they are a father, mother, husband, wife, child, sibling, grandparent, etc. to avoid embarrassment.

CHAPTER 7

Storytelling: joy that is contagious

"Laughter is the best medicine".

(Author unknown)

Each day as a storyteller represents a very joyful and fun learning opportunity, because in addition to being very pleasurable, since you always end the day better than you started, in an atmosphere of joy, good humour and relaxation, you take with you experiences and stories that would never be possible otherwise. This is because, as already said, bibliotherapy is a tool whose benefit occurs in all directions, for all involved.

Stories for adults

Stories told to adults should be motivational, reflective and sometimes humorous. Currently, the Storytellers Group has a collection of about 80 stories selected by the group, which are used throughout the year, one story per week. Drawn from a wide variety of sources, they always carry a positive message and are told with full intonation and interpretation by the members of the group, who put emotion and life into each of the words contained in the story.

Below is an example of one of the stories used:

<u>Don't listen to the pessimists</u>

Once upon a time there was a race of... puppies. The goal was to reach the top of a large tower. On the spot, a crowd was watching. Lots of people to cheer and cheer for them. The competition began.

As the crowd, deep down, did not believe that the puppies could reach the top of that tower, what was heard most often was: "What a pity! The puppies won't make it. They won't make it".

And the puppies began to give up. But there was one puppy who persisted and kept climbing towards the top. The crowd kept shouting: "Oh, what a shame! You won't make it". And the puppies were giving up, one by one, except for that other one, who continued calmly, although panting.

By the end of the competition, everyone had given up except him. Curiosity then took over everyone. They wanted to know what had happened.

And when they gathered round the winning puppy to ask him how he had managed to complete the race, they discovered that he was deaf.

(Reflection) Every day we are bombarded with negative words. Trust in your potential and work towards realising your dreams. Be positive. It will do you and others good.

Author unknown

Stories for children and adolescents

In the environment of public hospitals, where people aged 0 to 18 years are admitted to the paediatric ward, it is very common to find children of very different ages in the same room, despite the efforts of the staff to maintain homogeneity in the rooms.

The fact that up to four children cohabit in the same room can be seen positively, as a sense of community and collaboration takes over in this situation. The parents or carers of these children develop friendships with their roommates, and can talk, exchange information, help each other and be an important support for each other within the hospital during treatment.

Another factor that deserves attention is the time available. Taking into account all the movement that occurs with these children during a day of hospitalisation, such as exams, visits from doctors, nurses, physiotherapists, psychologists, nutritionists, relatives, one should not use an extensive part of their time with bibliotherapy, however much one believes in its potential benefits.

Paracelsus, a Swiss-German physician and physicist of the 16th century, said that the difference between medicine and poison is in the dose. Therefore, the time and the amount of stories to be told should be enough to enchant, amuse and entertain these children and adolescents, so that it really makes this important moment something magical and unique in their lives, showing the good side of books and reading, without being tiring and boring.

Thus, the task of telling stories in a playful and fun way to children in hospital should be done in such a way that the magic of bibliotherapy happens with the proper adaptation to the children's context. To this end, it is suggested that children's books be chosen according to the following practical criteria:

They are preferable:

- Stories with not too long text, so that the storyteller can learn and tell without the support of reading at the time of the activity;
- Books that have only illustrations, without text, so that the storyteller creates a story with or without the child's participation;
- Illustrations are very welcome, especially for babies;
- Mystery stories, superheroes, fairy tales, funny...;

30

- Books in 3D, with Pop-Ups and textures;
- Books that cater for a wide age range.
- Books that stimulate the imagination.

It is worth remembering that, in the case of bibliotherapy for children with some kind of illness, indisposition, or recovering in the home environment, these criteria are not fully applicable, since in this situation the freedom regarding time and activities is very variable, allowing a more personalised storytelling in which it is suggested that the books be chosen according to the profile and taste of the child or, if very small, of their guardians. There is also the possibility of using a single book for several days, counting a part or chapter per day.

Books used for children:

The ladybird - Collection of fun animals in 3D - various authors

Who let out the bam? - Blandina Franco and José Carlos Lollo

Even princesses can fart - Ilan Brenman

The cow that laid an egg - Russell Ayto

A monkey forwards - Ruth Rocha

The porridge bug - Paula Browne

Once upon a time there was a wolf Mingau - Alessandra Roscoe

The worm in love - Alessandra Roscoe

Time keeping box - Alessandra Roscoe

Selena: the indecisive snake - Kate Thomson

Witch: come to my party - Arden Druce

SpongeBob at: surprise party - Ciranda Cultural

Charades moment: Riddles for all

Riddles, charades and jokes are considered to be great helpers when the bibliotherapeutic process takes place, before or after the storytelling. Sometimes they are used before to get attention to the story or children's books. Other times they are used after the story, to cheer up and bring a little fun to the patient(s) and their companion(s). However, in all cases it is recommended to pay attention to the moment of the patient and to observe the appropriateness of the application of this tool.

What is what:

1. Who is born in RIO, lives in RIO, but is not always wet? Carioca.
2. A little red dot on top of the castle? Black pepper.

3. In the aquarium there are 10 fish, 5 drown, how many are left? 10, fish do not drown.

4. What's in the middle of the egg?"V"

5. What does the ant have that is bigger than the lion? Name.

6. A duck walks up a slope and lays an egg; does the egg go up or down? A duck does not lay an egg, it lays an egg with its duck.

7. Who is born big and dies small? Pencil.

8. What does the witch use to fly when it's raining? Squeegee.

9. What walks on its head? Louse.

10. What hits us, but we never complain? Heart.

11. It has a cat's tail, cat's eye, cat's ears, meows like a cat and is not a cat? Cat.

12. What makes a man turn his head? Neck.

13. What did the stamp say to the envelope? Stick it on me and let's go for a walk.

14. Do you sleep standing up and walk lying down? Standing.

15. What's a little black dot inside an aeroplane? An aeromosk.

16. Who has 7 lives but is not a cat? It's the cat.

17. What did the post say to the dog? There's no point in watering, I won't grow anymore.

18. What is born from the crossing of a giraffe and a parrot? A speaker.

19. How does a snake save a person from a flood? By striking.

20. What has a mouth but doesn't speak? The cooker.

21. Why does the ox go up the hill? Because it can't go under.

22. The cinema was full of cement, what was the name of the film? None, the cinema was under construction.

23. That the more you lose, the more you have? Sleep.

24. What did zero say to eight? What a cool belt!!!

25. Why does the madman shower with the shower off? Because he bought shampoo for dry hair.

26. What's the end of the bite? When the mosquito goes away.

27. That the more it grows the less you see? The darkness.

28. The more you wipe, the wetter it gets? Towel.

29. How many animals did Moses put in the ark? None, because it wasn't Moses who put them in, it was Noah.

30. Which animal eats with its bum? All of them! They can't take their tails out to eat!

31. What is the difference between an ox and a clown? The ox likes green straw and the clown likes clowning.

32. A hen climbed high in a tree to lay an egg, what did she say? Now I'm going to break it.

33. Which mobile phone operator has the flu? Tim.

34. How many sheep does it take to make a woollen coat? Just one, as long as she knows how to knit.

35. That breathes without lungs and has feet but does not walk? Tree.

36. What did one cockroach say to another? My boyfriend is a cockroach.

37. There are 7 siblings, 5 have a surname and 2 don't, which are? The days of the week.

38. What goes around all the time, but doesn't go anywhere? The hands of the clock.

39. What is good for walking, but doesn't go anywhere? The street.

Cumulus

What is the height of patience?
A: Watching the slug race in slow motion.

What is the height of amnesia?
A: Oh, I forgot.

What is the height of organisation?
A: Having alphabet soup.

What is the height of stupidity?
R1: Draw "even or odd" with the mirror and choose odd.
R2: Spy through the keyhole of a glass door.

What is the height of trust?
A: Playing hopscotch on the phone.

What is the height of sluggishness?
A: Betting a race alone and coming 2nd.

What is the height of laziness?
R1: Waking up earlier to spend more time doing nothing.
R2: Lie in the hammock and wait for the wind to sway.

What is the height of vision?

A: Take down 10 fighters with just one glancing blow.

What is the height of Selfishness?
A: I won't tell, only I know!

What is the height of ignorance?
A: Open the pen to find the little letters.

What is the height of exaggeration?
A: Buttering the sugar loaf.

What is the height of strength?
R1: Round the corner.
R2: Tie your trainers with a ship's anchor.

What is the height of speed?
R1: Go round the block and meet your back.
R2: Lock the drawer and put the key inside.

What is the pinnacle of basketball?
A: Throw the ball in the basket and hit Saturday.

What is the height of rebellion?
A: Living alone and running away from home.

What is the maths crunch?
A: Order an X-burger, eat the burger and calculate the X.

CHAPTER 8

Stories from the hospital: endless lessons

"Love your neighbour as yourself".

-- Jesus

True story 1:

One day we entered a paediatric ward. There was a woman there with a little girl about a year old on her lap. One of the volunteers remarked to the woman that the little girl looked very much like her, that she had "taken after" her mother. That was when the woman replied, very gently, that it was love that made the two look alike, as the little girl was her adopted daughter. Then she began to tell us about the congenital problem the child had and all the surgeries she had already undergone. Our surprise was great, but we had to contain our emotion to be able to continue the day's work, as this was the first room we had entered. We learnt that it is always better to control our curiosity, not to ask questions about kinship, not even indirectly, and to remember that we don't really need to know what the illness or treatment in question is, since our role is to make them forget, for a moment, what they are going through and transport them to the world of stories in which anything can happen. (Fabyola Lima Madeira)

True story 2:

We once entered a room where the patients were four elderly women. As we entered, one of them said she did not want to hear stories and turned her back to us in her bed. Meanwhile the others said they wanted to listen. So, with great humour and politeness, we said that we would then tell the story only to the others without any problem. At the end of the story, we talked a little and then we started the riddles, to relax and liven up the atmosphere, since the patients and carers were a little shy and did not talk much. As soon as we started, the patient who did not want to hear stories started to "kick" answers to the riddles even with her back turned, then she turned around and started to participate in the game, she laughed a lot with the answers to the riddles and with all the racket we made with each new question. In the end, she was the one who had the most fun and thanked us for being there. At that moment, we had yet another demonstration that the world of stories and riddles - which are still stories in the form of questions - is more seductive than you might think! (Fabyola

35

Lima Madeira)

True story 3:

"It was on a hot, dry September afternoon that I met Mrs Dalvina, who was hospitalised on the cardiology floor of the Hospital de Base. With a calm countenance, she appeared to be no more than forty years old. Only two teeth showed in her smile. Her clumsy hair was tied in a ponytail. She shared the room with three other patients and lively visitors. We, the Storytellers, received a warm welcome and narrated the plot of the disciple who went to consult the monk on how to deal with the faults of the people who annoyed him. The warning was clear: to worry about correcting his own faults and ignore those of others. A beautiful fable about acceptance.

The success was immediate, but unlike the other rooms, there the message of unconditional acceptance of the human being would not come from the story, but from the calm and simple Mrs Dalvina, who told us a little about her daily life where she lives, on the outskirts of the city. She told us that, despite the warnings of her neighbours, she always leaves the door of her house open. Among the people who visit her daily is a boy who takes drugs, commits crimes and frightens the neighbourhood. She does not know why, but he comes to her every day.

- I let him in and he asks me for money. I say: I don't have money, but I'll give him food. He stays there and doesn't say anything. The next day, I say: Give up this life of drugs. You know what happens to those who get into that life, right? They die.

The whole room is silent. She continues:

- But I don't judge him. I know that if I do that, he'll go away and, while he's there, I'll find a way to talk to him. Do you know that after a while he really gave up drugs? He told me he was going back to school. Can you imagine if I had fought with him?

In a violent and harsh world, Dona Dalvina distributes hope and consideration. And because she always leaves her front door open, there's more to the story:

- The other day a woman came in who had just been shot in the leg. She came asking for water and I said: I won't give you water. You can go away because you won't get any water here. The neighbours arrived, everyone terrified by the scene, the woman bleeding and asking for water for God's sake. I turned to my neighbour, who was going to get a glass of water for the woman, and told her she was crazy, that if I gave her water she would die right there.

I didn't understand, I asked why I couldn't give water and Mrs Dalvina explained that if the girl had an internal haemorrhage and took water she would die on the spot. Mrs Dalvina knew about medicine. The silence with which everyone in the room listened to her was giving the dimension of our true size before that patient. There was no degree of study or self-knowledge that would bring us even a little closer to the giant Mrs Dalvina. Without prejudice or judgement, she had no fear. Without fear,

36

she lived the fullness of a clear conscience. In the midst of difficulties and violence, she did not refuse help, but did so with the respect and care to which every human being is entitled.

If we are just starting to accept people, trying to judge the other in a less ruthless and prejudiced way, trying to make our personal relationships more friendly, opening our minds to other ways of life different from ours, there are people like Mrs Dalvina who opens the door of her house and welcomes anyone. She has no money to give, but love overflows in the simple attitude of denying a glass of water to those who cannot take it and in the respect she has for even the worst marginal.

It was another afternoon when we left the hospital with the feeling that true learning is where it is least expected. That we are light years away from the wisdom and purity of a simple Mrs Dalvina, who does not need to read to experience the humility and welcome that we so much seek. That afternoon, I felt like a repeating student in front of a renowned teacher". (Ana Cristina Sampaio Alves)

CHAPTER 9

Experience reports: each person a story

"Start by doing what's necessary, then what's possible, and suddenly you'll be doing the impossible".

St Francis of Assisi

"To say what the job of storyteller represents for me at the same time is an easy task, because of the love I feel, but very difficult to be expressed in words. First of all, this work is for me a possibility and opportunity to love! Not love for those we already love, which we always try to practise, but selfless love for a complete stranger, to whom I can give my time, my attention, my smile and my gaze! And how beautiful it is to see the receptivity of all this by our patients and carers! The smiles received in return, as well as the attentive looks, or the prayers that are made to us, by practitioners of the most diverse creeds, out of gratitude, or simply the tears of emotion that are shed by those who listen to us, and who still apologise for it, believe me?! And how they teach us! How many times I arrive at the beds thinking that I am going to donate... and I hear incredible life stories, of warrior and inspiring people, who even in pain manage to smile (with their lips and with their eyes)... that's when I realise that I get much more in return. And if you imagine that at some point the activity becomes tedious, repetitive, make no mistake! Every day is completely different from the other, and even if we are telling the same story, to the same ward, we can always get something better out of it, for us and for the next! Telling stories for me is a fulfilment, it's reframing and giving purpose to my life, it's always learning and growing! And one thing we often say in the group is that if we tell the same story several times in the same day, we are hearing it several times too, most probably because we are the ones who need it the most".

Daniel Novais (Storytelling Group volunteer and Saturday team coordinator)

"My life has always been about reading and telling stories. Since I was a child, I used to write novels and read them to my mum in the kitchen. They were stories of witches, abandoned girls, castles and princesses.

Later, as a journalist, I began to narrate true events. But my first experience as a storyteller in hospital came when my sister, who died aged 11, was hospitalised for a month. During that time, I read to her daily.

38

Perhaps it was because I was so familiar with storytelling that storytelling struck me as the perfect volunteer job. As I often say to newcomers and those interested: it is so simple that you only need to be literate to do it.

However, reading to patients is a task that surprises by its transformative potential, not only of your soul, but of those you reach with the interpretation of the story.

At first, every story I told seemed to have been written directly to me. How was it possible that a fable could tell me so many truths at once? It was as if my entire emotional cache came to the surface in those simple, yet deeply philosophical and reflective narratives.

After each afternoon of storytelling, I would have a coffee with myself, as if to digest the teachings I had read to simple people, but who with each comment showed me how much they were learning from the disease.

Thus began my transformation in the task. And I, who until recently could not even smell a hospital, started to talk to amputees, victims of accidents and violence, heart patients, haemophiliacs, neurosurgery patients, people with cancer and other serious illnesses, and even to the prisoners in Papuda who needed hospitalisation.

Needless to say, it wasn't just the stories handpicked by the group coordinators to allow for light-hearted conversation on deep topics, the socialising with fellow storytellers, or the difficult scenes I witnessed in the countless rooms I visited that made me a different person in such a short time. What made a decisive and inexorable contribution to my change was getting to know the reality behind the disease. It is impossible to spend five years in hospitals telling stories and come out of the experience unscathed. The contact with the life of each patient and their family, who listen to the narrative and participate in it animatedly, allows us to exchange feelings and emotions so particular, so often unconscious and unknown, that we are drawn into a new vision of life.

The personal transformation of a storyteller happens in a joyful, humorous way, sometimes intense by contact with a more painful experience, but with generous doses of reality, such as overcoming, persistence, patience and acceptance. Each year we retell an old story, but it is already different. The interpretation of the group, the direction of the conversation that follows is always new and vibrant. In each room, a different reality. Otherness at its highest level. That is why every storyteller who remains in hospital is destined to become someone who moves between the imaginary and the concrete, the cold word and the emotion, while learning to cultivate hope, good cheer, faith in the future and health above all."

Ana Cristina Sampaio Alves (Storytelling Group volunteer)

"The importance of storytellers at Hospital de Base is enormous, especially in this digital

age. When they arrive with their crazy hats, huge glasses, and their different voices, they already catch the attention of the children, and they manage to awaken both the little ones and the parents the magic of listening to a good story. As a teacher I see the good they bring, not only for the joy they share, but for helping us to open the doors of this wonderful world, which is reading, making them forget, for a while, where they are and easing some of the suffering".

Crishna Morelo

Hospital class teacher at Instituto Hospital de Base

"My story began after hearing another story. It was in a course, whose theme was apparently unrelated, that I learnt, through the account of one of the participants, about the work done by the Storytellers at the Hospital de Base de Brasília. I joined them, both out of a desire/duty to help others and to spend some time with the children, at a time when I saw my dream of becoming a mother so far from reality.

It was 4 years of much love, stories and stories, until I had to move away to finally take care of the being that God entrusted especially to me. Dream realised! And during all this time, I realised that the cliché - in volunteer work we receive more than we give - is the purest truth. Storytelling is a two-way therapy, hand in hand, an infinite exchange of energies. It is magical to see the power that a few words, a few drawings and a little goodwill have to change people's mood.

I could see children dragging their IV stands through the hospital corridors to follow, from door to door, the stories that were told next to the beds... corridors that were also the stage for many stories, destined for a single person bored of staying in their room or for an audience that just wanted to share... stories that were almost always repeated, but that gained new life when they were told to different children, with different trajectories and destinies, or to the same children, but on different days, with experiences never lived before.

I could see parents entertaining themselves more than their children, recovering memories of their childhoods and letting the laughter explode on their faces, relieving the tensions of a heart so distressed at the time. And when that child who plays hide-and-seek among the accumulating years is found, we strip ourselves of all fear, prejudice and judgement, to just, and so intensely, surrender to the stories.

I could see denials and withdrawals turn into interest, willingness and joy. And how many times were these same children, previously apathetic, who asked for an encore. They, and so many others, wanted more... more fantasy, more lightness in their days, more attention, more ears even... and storytellers are also listeners... of those individuals who want to be the protagonists of their own stories, whether with a simple "aunt, I have a little white dog with black spots" or with the whole

40

long, complex and beautiful narrative about Asdrubal and his watch.... about the appreciation of time... about living intensely every second... for me, particularly, the most exciting and striking moment of all, the story told with perfection and much joy by a soul who had to, from an early age, learn to read the world through other eyes.

This outstanding chapter, however, in no way diminishes all the other experiences, lessons and feelings planted, cultivated, blossomed and harvested in the paediatrics department of Hospital de Base. Stories of life and for life. Stories that will always be balm and motivation for listening hearts and also tellers. Eternal gratitude for this opportunity! "

Monica Barreiro da Costa (Storytellers Group volunteer)

"Once upon a time, I really wanted to do voluntary work, but I kept thinking to myself: I don't know how to sew or make crafts, I can't cook, I can't teach or do anything special. How could I do such a job?

One day I found out that there was a Storytellers group. I was happy and decided to give it a try, but deep down inside, a doubt assailed me. What difference would it make to tell a story to an adult hospital patient? What would it change for them? What benefit would it bring?

I started the job. I would find out and it was love at first sight. At first, I realised that it is easy to tell stories, you just need to know how to read well and be willing to help. Then, I found a lot of affection in those who listen to us and a very positive feedback from them about the storytelling. The doubts disappeared. The patients revealed to me that a little attention and affection can change the day and, perhaps, someone's life. That a smile sweetens the day. That the exchange of an experience can lead us to rethink what we are and what we do. That reflections sometimes reveal a new path for those who no longer see the direction. That a little distraction and fun can make a painful moment lighter.

And it was in this way, with this exchange that we have with them every week, that I found many answers. I'm still finding them. That's how I managed to fill this space that was blank inside me. A space that now has colours, presences, sounds and smiles. "

Arlana Fernandes Azevedo (Storytellers Group volunteer)

CHAPTER 10

The power of stories as mental reprogramming

"Every good deed you do is a light you create around your own steps."

Chico Xavier

The positive impact caused by an experience such as Bibliotherapy, in which most of the senses (sight, hearing, smell, speech) are extremely activated from the beginning of the story until the possible dialogue that follows, is capable of promoting a mental reprogramming in the individuals who participate in it. This type of experience can be considered one of the most complete in terms of absorption of knowledge and expansion of consciousness to new possibilities, due to the very natural way in which it develops. What proves the effectiveness of activities of this nature is NLP (Neurolinguistic Programming).

According to Robbins (2017, 28 ed., p. 248), "*one of the best ways to become aware of the amazing diversity of human reactions is to talk to a group of people. You can't help but notice how differently people react to the same thing. You tell a motivational story and one person is amazed, while another finds it dull. You tell a joke, and one person laughs, while another doesn't move a muscle. You think that each person is listening in a different mental language.*"

When a story is told that is commonly used in bibliotherapy, and usually carries some kind of implicit positive reflection or message, the listener is given the opportunity to hear it and come to their own conclusions. The narrators fulfil the role of making a caring, light and loving approach, so that the participants feel welcomed and at ease so that the storytelling can begin. This preparation of the listeners aims to make them more receptive to the experience, while the preparation of the environment aims to create a quiet, relaxed and pleasant atmosphere. This set of actions is considered fundamental to the success of the story as a form of mental reprogramming.

The mental programming to which a sick person may be subject, sometimes extremely detrimental to their treatment or recovery, is totally linked to their inner beliefs and representations, stemming from the experiences and facts that make up their past or even from stories they have heard. These inner representations and beliefs direct the person's life, enabling them to make choices and to form an internal list of the possibilities they accept. These possibilities may be very limited, making life and consequently the individual's treatment or recovery difficult.

42

According to NLP, internal representations are structured through the five senses, so that whatever experiences are stored in the mind are represented through these senses, but mainly through the three major modalities: visual, auditory and kinaesthetic. Thus, some people are more visual, so they perceive the world and its messages predominantly through images or what they see; other people are more auditory, reacting to stimuli to a greater degree by what they hear; and others are more kinaesthetic, understanding messages according to what they feel.

The mental programmes can be represented by the feelings that emanate, because the experiences stored in the subconscious memory of the individual have varied vibrational frequencies: high are positive and low are negative (according to Fig.1). These feelings remain alive, vibrating in the subject's body field as long as that programming exists, generating more of that in his life. Some examples of feelings that people in a situation of illness may present: victimisation, fear, revolt, anger, indignation, hurt, rejection, sadness, disappointment, despair, anxiety.

As science proves that like attracts like, the power of bibliotherapy lies in bringing stories that deconstruct negative beliefs, promote mental reprogramming with positive stories, expand the consciousness of those who listen and thus start to vibrate at higher frequencies. With this, the old negative feelings are replaced by more beneficial ones, putting an end to the eternal *looping of* undesirable situations. Examples of positive emotions are: faith, self-confidence, worthiness, self-love, acceptance, joy, happiness. Through this change, mental patterns also change and healing becomes something very natural.

If a person believes that something is impossible and suddenly hears a story in which that situation was possible, making him completely change his paradigm, that person has undergone a mental reprogramming, he has expanded his consciousness, which is why he now sees more possibilities than before. In addition, her list of beliefs has changed and what she believes shapes her reality. This simple change can fill a person with hope, joy, optimism, confidence and this in many cases is enough to heal, this is the role of bibliotherapy.

References

SEITZ, Eva Maria. **Bibliotherapy**: an experience with patients hospitalised in a medical clinic. Florianópolis: Habitus, 2006.

VASQUEZ, Maria do Socorro Azevedo Felix Fernandez. **Bibliotherapy for the elderly**: a case study in the Providence Home "Carneiro da Cunha", 1989. Dissertation (master's degree in Library Science) - Centre for Applied Social Sciences, Federal University of Paraíba.

ALVES, Maria Helena Hees. A aplicação da biblioterapia no processo de reintegração social. **Revista Brasileira de Biblioteconomia e Documentação**, v. 15, n. 1/2, jan./jun. 1982.

CALDIN, Clarice Fortkamp. **Bibliotherapy**: a care with the being. São Paulo: Porto de Ideias, 2010. 199 p.

CASTRO, Rachel; PINHEIRO, Edna. **Bibliotherapy for the elderly**: what remains and what it means. Biblionline, v. 1, n. 2,2005. Available at: http://periodicos.ufpb.br/ojs2/index.php/biblio/article/viewFile/586/424 Accessed on: 1 July 2018.

CHOPRA, Depack. **The quantum cure**. 48. ed. Rio de Janeiro: BestSeller, 2013.

HOSPITAL DE BASE, a health heritage to be preserved: an X-ray of the largest medical centre in the Federal District. **Rev. Médico em dia. May/Jun. 2017.** p. 23-27.

MAP OF CONSCIOUSNESS . Available at : <https://institutotaiyoo.wordpress.com/2017/07/15/voce-sabia-que-cada-sentimento- energy-what-you-vibrate-can-be-measured-and-what-it-influences-in-your-destination/> Accessed: 20 May 2018.

Robbins, Anthony. **Awaken your inner giant**: how to take control of everything in your life. 33. ed. Rio de Janeiro: BestSeller, 2017. 615 p.

Robbins, Anthony. **Power without limits**. 28. ed. Rio de Janeiro: BestSeller, 2017. 404 p.

Agenda 2030
Available at: <http://www.agenda2030.org.br/sobre/> Accessed on: 1 Aug. 2018.

Brazilian Congress of Library, Documentation and Information Science: Libraries and the 2030 Agenda
Available at: <https://www.cbbd2017.com/trabalhos> Accessed on: 1 Aug. 2018.

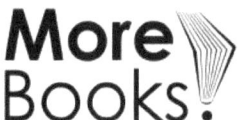
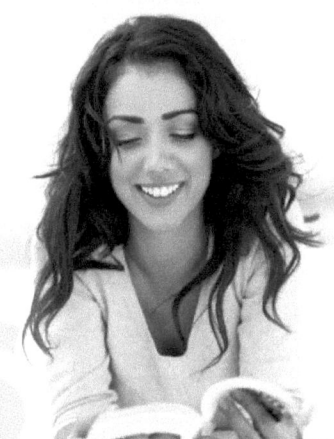

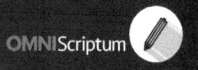

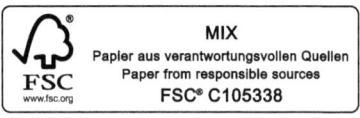
Printed by Books on Demand GmbH, Norderstedt / Germany